HOLISTIC CHILDBIRTH MANUAL

AN INCLUSIVE, HOLISTIC, EVIDENCE BASED CHILDBIRTH GUIDE

JACKY BLOEMRAAD-DE BOER, MIDWIFE, L.AC., NUTRITIONIST

Copyright © 2023 by Jacky Bloemraad-de Boer

All rights reserved.

No portion of this book may be reproduced in any form without written permission from the publisher or author, except as permitted by U.S. copyright law.

Cover image by Faraz Ahmed @ Fiverr.com

"In giving birth to our babies, we find that we give birth to new possibilities within ourselves." ~ Myla Kabat-Zinn

Contents

1. Authors Note — 1
2. APGAR — 3
3. Baby's Position during Birth — 6
4. Caesarean (C-section) — 11
5. Contractions — 26
6. Continuity of care — 30
7. Delayed (optimal) Cord Clamping — 33
8. Dilation — 36
9. Engagement of the baby's head — 38
10. Eating & Drinking during labour — 40
11. Episiotomy — 43
12. Foetal Monitoring in Labour — 46
13. Hormones of Labour and birth — 48
14. Induction of Labour — 55

15.	Inviting Labour naturally	64
16.	Labour	70
17.	Mucous Plug	81
18.	Managing Labour Pain	83
19.	Medical pain relief	89
20.	Nutritional Preparation for Labour and birth	95
21.	Positions for Labour and Birth	101
22.	Premature Labour	106
23.	Placenta (the birth of)	107
24.	Vaginal Examinations	111
25.	VBAC	114
26.	Waterbirth	118

About Author	120
Also By	121
Bonus Material	123
References and Research	124

Authors Note

This A-Z formatted manual strives to prepare women for an optimal childbirth experience. Giving evidence-based information, empirical knowledge and holistic recommendations about what you can do to promote this physiological process.

It doubles up as a handy reference pocket for both parents and professionals working in the field of childbirth. It covers the physiological process of childbirth, the importance of understanding the essential cocktail of birth hormones, ways that women can find solace during labour and birth, the role of pain, the various terms used during and around childbirth, and the importance of continuous emotional and physical support. The specific advice given can (and should be) adapted in a way that is culturally appropriate for each family.

I have adapted my texts in certain places for the language to be more inclusive without excluding the traditional language of women or motherhood. When I use the terms "woman/women and mothers" I am referring to sex as a reproductive category versus gender as a societal role or gender identity.

> *A woman's childbirth experience is vitally important, and there is enough to show that women's birthing memories endure. The major factors that influence the quality of a woman's birth experience include personal expectations, the quality and amount of support she receives, the quality of the caregiver-patient relationship - specifically communication, continuity of care, empathy, and respect, - her involvement in decision making, her clinical risk and outcome.*

APGAR

An APGAR score is used to assess your baby's basic condition at the time of birth. It is named after Virginia Apgar and is also an acronym for the things that are checked and observed.

The score of the test is a total of 10 with each aspect being scored from zero to two and are done at ONE and again at FIVE minutes. If there are concerns, the APGAR may be done again at TEN minutes intervals.

A

Appearance (Colour) If the baby's entire body is pale or blue all over, a score of 0 is given. Babies whose bodies are pinkish but who have blue extremities or a blue face are awarded a score of one. There are not many occurrences that the baby's colour is such that it receives a score of two.

P

Pulse (Heart rate) The heart rate is the baby's pulse. If there is no pulse at all, a score of zero is given. A slow pulse, a score of one is given. A pulse of more than 100 bpm (beats per minute) would receive a score of two.

G

Grimace (Reflex irritability) This assessment is made by stimulating the baby, either by drying it, talking to it, rubbing its back or the soles of its feet. If there is no reaction or response then the score is zero. Some grimace or reaction results in the score of one. If the baby cries, coughs, sneezes or grimaces then the score that is given is two.

A

Activity (Muscle Tone) This assessment is done by looking at the movement of the baby. A baby that is not moving or is 'floppy' would be given a score of zero. A baby that was moving its limbs in a minimal way receives a score of 1. Babies that are active with good tone in their limbs are given a score of two.

R

Respiratory Effort (Breathing) This relates to the ability of the baby to breathe. If at 1-minute the baby is not breathing, the score would be zero. A slow respiratory rate, irregular breathing, or difficulty breathing, receives a score of one. A normal respiratory rate with no abnormal effort, or a baby that is crying normally, receives a score of two.

APGAR results

A baby who scores **seven** or above at ***ONE minute*** after birth is considered to be in good health. However, a lower score doesn't necessarily mean that your baby is unhealthy or abnormal. For example, a score between four and six at one minute indicates that your baby needs more time to adjust or they sometimes just need some aid/assistance to take their first breath.

At **FIVE minutes** after birth, the Apgar score is re-calculated and if your baby's score hasn't improved to seven or greater, your care provider will continue any necessary medical care and will closely monitor your baby.

Baby's Position during Birth

At the onset and during labour and birth there are more favourable and less favourable positions for the baby to be in.

Favourable Position: when most babies enter the pelvis head down, the baby's chin is tucked in touching his chest. This position helps the crown of the baby's head to enter the pelvis first so the head can mould to fit through the pelvis. The skull of a baby isn't fused, so the bones can shift (mould), to allow them to fit through the birth canal.

During birth the most favourable position for your baby to be moving through your pelvis is head-down with the back of his head towards your front, this is called an anterior position. Labour tends to be shorter and easier in comparison to a baby that is in a posterior position - see below. In an anterior position, your baby fits snugly into the curve of your pelvis and it's easier for them to move down, into and through your pelvis during labour.

Less Favourable Position/s: some babies move down into the pelvis with the back of their head towards their mother's spine. This is called a posterior position or a back-to-back position. We tend to see longer labours with more difficulties and complications when a baby is in a posterior position - especially in first births. A baby in a posterior position cannot tuck its chin to its chest which means that the top of the head is entering the pelvis rather than the crown. The top of the head is a larger surface and it does not mould as well as the crown. The baby's spine is also extended rather than curled, which also prevents the crown from entering the pelvis first.

Posterior position difficulties/complications:

- Possible longer pregnancy.
- The amniotic sac breaking (water breaks/rupture of membranes) before labour (1 in 5 posterior labours).
- Labour is longer and stronger and less rhythmic than expected.
- Start and stop labour pattern.
- The baby may not engage, even during the pushing stage.
- Back labour (in many cases).
- Longer pushing stage.
- Sometimes the baby's head gets jammed because of the larger leading circumference.
- More likely to tear.

- More likely to need a vacuum (ventouse) or forceps.
- More likely to need a C-section.

Babies will try to find the position in which they feel more comfortable in the uterus. For the baby to adopt an anterior position the mother's front needs to feel like a comfortable hammock. To support this, the mother's main positions in the last weeks of pregnancy and then during labour should be forward-leaning ones.

When a pregnant woman sits down for long periods (at a desk or in a car) or leans back, as she reclines with her feet up after a long day, the baby will feel most comfortable lying on his mother's back.

If women have a lifestyle that involves very little sitting and a lot of upright activities their baby is far more likely to go down into your pelvis in an anterior position because their pelvis is often tipped more forwards.

Helping your baby into an anterior position before birth

Helping your baby to move into an anterior rather than a posterior position is called "optimal foetal positioning". You can encourage your baby to take up this optimal position by making sure that you don't spend all day sitting and when you do sit, ensure you don't slump into a "hammock shape" for your baby to lie in towards your back. Don't put your feet up; lying back with your feet up encourages posterior presentation. If you spend a long time watching television try to sit with a straight back and move onto hands and knees, rocking your pelvis from side to side for at least five minutes every 20 minutes. Reclining (hanging) forward over a birthing ball, the back of the couch or a chair can invite the baby to swivel forward into the "hammock-shape" you are creating by doing this.

Improving the baby's position during labour

The best thing you can do during labour to help your baby position more favourably is to change your position regularly, avoid lying on your back or being immobile for too long.

Move the Mother to Move the Baby

Regularly changing positions will have a positive influence on the labour process.

Keeping in mind that you should change into a new position every 30 to 40 minutes, here are some positions you could try:

- Kneel with pillows (for comfort) under your hands and knees.

- Walk around slowly or stand leaning forward onto a surface and rock your pelvis from side to side.

- Walk up and down stairs (slowly and sideways if you need to). This can help the baby to re-position in your pelvis.

- Step on and off a small stool.

- If you get very tired during labour, lie on your left side with a chinky pillow between your knees as this gives your baby some space while you are resting.

> *The very best advice I can give on this subject is to head over to the Spinning Babies website during pregnancy to benefit from all the helpful information about your body comfort during pregnancy and on how to optimise your baby's position before going into labour:* https://www.spinningbabies.com

Caesarean (C-section)

The term Caesarean section or C-section refers to the operation that delivers a baby through incisions made in the mother's abdominal wall and uterus. It remains one of medicine's most important and often lifesaving operations. However, a planned Caesarean delivery without a medical reason (indication) has not been proven to reduce any risk to either mother or baby and it has been proven to increase complications during the delivery and postpartum period for both the mother and the baby.

Valid reasons for a scheduled C-section

• If the placenta is blocking the exit of the uterus (placenta previa.)

• If there is a history of uterine surgery or abnormalities.

• Rarely, diabetes mellitus or hypertension can threaten the baby's welfare which creates an acute need for the baby to be delivered.

• When anatomical problems of the uterus or birth canal prevent successful vaginal birth.

When a C-section is scheduled there is the possibility of requesting a **"Gentle" C-section.** With some prior planning with participating care providers and hospitals, assuming both you and the baby are doing well, you can request a gentle C-section. In a gentle C-section, the surgery remains the same, the difference is that efforts are made to personalise the experience.

For example, lights may be dimmed, music may be played, the drape that normally obscures the mom's view of the operation may be clear, and once the baby's head is out of the abdomen, the rest of the body is brought out slower (this can help to squeeze out fluid from the baby's lungs) and skin-to-skin contact with your baby immediately after the birth is prioritised.

Reasons for an unscheduled C-section

There is a difference between an unscheduled C-section and an emergency C-section, although people often use the terms interchangeably. Unplanned cesareans are still considered urgent, but typically mother and baby aren't in life-threatening situations.

Common causes for an urgent, unplanned C-section during labour could include:

- Labour fails to progress after a certain amount of hours with contractions and/or pushing without progress
- Labour induction fails
- The baby isn't tolerating labour

- The baby is lying sideways (transverse) when labour begins

Maternal or foetal emergencies that require an emergency C-section:

- Untimely separation of the placenta from the uterus

- An active vaginal infection of herpes or a life-threatening bacterial infection

- If the umbilical cord drops into the birth canal ahead of the baby, which is referred to as a prolapsed umbilical cord

- Any indication that the baby would be better off out of the womb than in it

- A baby that has compromised health and will not be able to endure labour contractions

More than one-fifth of all births are by C-section, and roughly only one-fifth of all C-section deliveries are prompted by an emergency condition.

Anaesthetic

There are 3 types of anaesthetic you may be given so that you do not feel any pain during your operation:

They include:

- **Spinal anaesthetic** – the most common anaesthetic for a planned caesarean. A needle will be inserted between the bones in your spine and local anaesthetic will be injected through the needle. This will block the pain from your chest downwards. You will be awake and able to breathe normally. As your baby is being born, you may feel tugging and pulling sensations, but no pain. In some cases, a pain-killing medicine (morphine) is given at the same time as the spinal. This can last for the next 24 hours and helps with your recovery as you are less drowsy and able to eat, drink and walk around earlier. Ask your doctor if this is offered at your hospital.

- **Epidural anaesthetic** is often used to lessen the pain of labour. If you have already been given an epidural during labour, and it is working well, the epidural can be topped up for an emergency caesarean. The epidural is a plastic tube that will be inserted into a space around the lining of your spine. Local anaesthetic will be injected through the tube, which will block any pain sensation from your waist down. You will be awake and able to breathe normally. As your baby is being born, you may feel tugging and pulling sensations, but no pain.

- **A general anaesthetic** may also be given if your baby needs to be born very quickly. You will breathe oxygen through a mask and you will be given medicine through a drip, which will make you drowsy and put you to sleep. You will sleep through your baby's birth.

The C-section Procedure

- A urinal catheter will be placed

- You are placed on an operating table, which may be slightly tilted

- A screen is placed so you cannot see the operation being done

- Once you are anaesthetised the doctor makes a cut in your lower abdomen, just above your pubic bone and then a cut in your uterus - both about 10 cm long

- When the doctor reaches the uterus, you may hear suctioning. After cutting through the uterus, the amniotic fluid will be suctioned away

- Your baby's head will be lifted out through the incision. Sometimes the doctor may use forceps to help lift out your baby's head

- Once the head is out, your doctor will suction the baby's nose and mouth for fluids. In a vaginal birth, these are squeezed out by the constriction of labour. In a cesarean birth, the baby needs some extra help getting rid of these fluids

- Once your baby has been suctioned, the doctor will start to help the rest of the body to be born. The doctor will need to manoeuvre the baby back and forth to help them emerge

- The doctor will check for umbilical cord entanglement or other complications as the body is born

- Your baby will be lifted up for you to see as soon as they have been delivered

- Your baby will be checked

- You will be able to hold your baby soon afterwards. Skin-to-skin contact can strengthen your early bond with your baby and make breastfeeding easier

- If you cannot hold your baby in the operating theatre, your support person will most likely be able to hold your baby instead

- The umbilical cord will be cut and your placenta will be removed

- An injection will be given to make your uterus contract and to minimise bleeding

- Antibiotics will be given to reduce the risk of infection

- The layers of muscle, fat and skin will be stitched back together and a dressing will be applied over the wound

GOOD TO KNOW INFORMATION ABOUT A C-SECTION

During the C-section

When having a spinal or epidural, even though you will not have any feeling in your lower body; you will feel the tugging and the pressure of the doctors at work to get your baby out.

Not only do you lose the ability to move from the chest down, but your arms are also immobilised so that you are perfectly still. Once your baby is born, the anaesthesiologist might free an arm so you can hug and touch your baby.

The entire process of removing your baby can take less than five minutes but then the remainder of the operation where they need to round off and then suture the abdomen can last anything from half an hour to an hour. Once the doctor has checked the baby, you or your partner may be able to hold the baby while the doctor manually removes your placenta, checks your uterus and sutures the incisions closed.

After the C-Section

Skin-to-Skin as soon as possible

If all went smoothly with you and baby then make sure to insist that your baby stays skin-to-skin with you as soon as possible and that it stays that way for as long as possible. Initiate breastfeeding as soon as possible. If the baby cannot be skin-to-skin with the mother then it should be skin-to-skin with her partner.

Take your pain killing meds around the clock for the first 48 hours.

It is recommended to take the daily dose of pain medication for the first couple of days at least to maintain the good levels in your bloodstream - this makes the medication more effective.

As a side note, while pain medication will let you focus on bonding with your new baby, they may have some side effects like constipation and nausea.

You will feel worse the second day

By day two your adrenaline and anything they gave you during your procedure will have worn off. Don't be surprised if you wake up on day two feeling more sore and tired than you did on day one. You may also experience more swelling than you did on the first day. All of this is normal but make sure to communicate any concerns to your nurse or doctor.

You'll still have postpartum bleeding

All mothers bleed after birth. You will need good sized maternity pads for the first two weeks. Women usually lose about 500ml during vaginal birth and around 1,000ml after a C-section.

Things you can't do for at least six weeks

You may be surprised to find that there are a lot of things your doctor will recommend you skip in those first six weeks until they can check your healing progress at your six-week postpartum checkup. Some restrictions are no driving or having sex, no heavy lifting, no using tampons and minimise taking the stairs.

You are allowed to be upset if your birth didn't go as planned / wished for

It's natural to spend your pregnancy imaging just how the day your child is born will play out. It's equally as natural to be upset if it doesn't end up anything as you'd envisioned.

Having a C-section doesn't disqualify you from having a vaginal birth in the future

If you plan to have another baby you should know that having one Caesarean birth doesn't mean future babies will require having one. Vaginal birth after a C-section, or VBAC for short, is not uncommon.

The success of a VBAC will depend on your preparation and the care provider that you choose

Go to the VBAC chapter for more information ->
#chapter=GSmpX0fMG69KW4Zq

Up and moving

Most women should begin walking within a day of their Caesarean delivery when a urinary catheter is no longer necessary. You can usually start eating a soft diet on the day after the operation, and you'll probably leave the hospital approximately 3 days after delivery. During your recovery, you may have to use a stool softener and a mild pain reliever. You will probably need to visit your doctor 2 to 3 weeks after leaving the hospital so he or she can examine your incision and remove any sutures or staples.

Planned Caesarean – the risks

If you are thinking of having a planned Caesarean delivery because you think it will be safer and less painful you might want to remember that a C-section is major abdominal surgery that carries risks.

Risks to you

- The risk of possible surgical complications such as the accidental cutting of your bladder or other internal organs

- Twenty percent chance you will get an infection as a result of the surgery.

- More blood loss - possibly resulting in a blood transfusion, higher risk of postpartum anaemia and PMAD.

- Higher risk of blood clots.

- Problems in future pregnancies such as low-lying placenta, placenta accreta (when it doesn't detach after birth and needs to be surgically removed. and damage to the wall of the uterus.

- Higher risk of bladder infection because you will have had a urinal catheter for during the operation and the first part of postpartum you have a higher risk of contracting a bladder infection

- More difficulty breastfeeding because of medication and due to the stress an operation has on your body it may take longer for the milk to come in. Also, the baby's instincts (reflexes) may be a little slow and it may take a while for it to "wake up".

Risks to the baby

- There is about a five per cent chance that when the surgeon cuts into your body during a Caesarean section, the knife will accidentally cut your baby.

- Because all the water is not squeezed out of the baby's lungs as is normally done during vaginal birth, more babies born after Caesarean section develop respiratory distress syndrome, which is a very serious newborn condition.

- Regularly, a Caesarean section is done too soon, because of the schedule of either the obstetrician or the mother, resulting in premature birth.

- Babies born via a choice C-section (when there have been no labour contractions to prepare the baby for birth) are known to have more digestive problems, more lung problems and more difficulty in breastfeeding.

When to consult your care provider postpartum after having a C- section

- If you develop a fever

- If you become dizzy or faint

- If you experience nausea and vomiting

- If you become short of breath

- If you have pain, swelling and redness at the incision site

- If you think you have a urinary tract infection

C-Section Preparation and Recovery Tips

1. Digestion

After a caesarean section, it is normal to feel nauseous, bloated and constipated, largely due to the pain medication and anaesthetic. It is best to wait until the bowels have "woken up" - one way to know this has happened is that you pass wind (fart) as soon as the bowel starts working again. Before this happens, it is best to eat small amounts of easily digestible food and drink only water.

The combination of lack of exercise, painkillers, antibiotics and the operation cause constipation and flatulence after the caesarean section.

What best to eat

Fibrous foods such as fruit, vegetables, whole grains, nuts, seeds and legumes, "mucilage forming" foods such as oats, chia and flaxseed. Liquid foods such as soups, stews, yoghurts and smoothies. Fermented vegetables such as sauerkraut or kimchi to aid digestion.

For bloating, add cardamom and ginger in your smoothies, drink them as herbal tea and liberally use them in cooking.

Water (about 8 glasses a day) - or according to thirst.

Herbs

Marshmallow Root (Althaea officinalis), 4 teaspoons in 1 litre of *cold* water and let steep for 1 hour.

Dosage: 1 cup every 4 hours

Nausea after a caesarean is incredibly common as a result of medication and as a stress reaction to surgery. Take Sea Band wristbands and ginger tea with you to the hospital.

Supplement

Probiotics - taken before and after the operation.

Antibiotics during/after caesarean section require supplementation of the good bacteria.

Important for: your immune system prevents common side effects like urinary tract infections and fungal infections.

Ensure that the baby gets probiotics through the breast milk.

Dosage:

Supplement with 10 to 20 billion colony forming units (CFU) - follow dosage advice of product.

EXTRA: Studies show that Lactobacillus rhamnosus HN001 administered during pregnancy and after childbirth can reduce depression and anxiety

2. Wound Healing

The wound needs 6-10 weeks to heal.

Expose to air for a few hours a day.

Use only water to clean the wound - dry well by dabbing.

Herbs

St. John's wort oil

Studies show that topical St. John's Wort oil improves healing.

Start on day 4.

Supplement

Glutamine has powerful effects on the immune system, muscles and tissue healing - all important after a caesarean.

Dosage:

0.5 g L-Glutamine per kg body weight.

Food sources of L-Glutamine: Bone broth, beef, spirulina, Chinese cabbage, whole cheese, whole yoghurt, spinach, asparagus, broccoli, wild caught fish (cod and salmon), wild poultry, turkey, eggs and nuts.

3. Nutrition for General Recovery

Bone broth for cell repair.

Iron-rich foods to counteract blood loss: red meat, seafood, egg yolks, oysters, dark leafy vegetables, nuts, seeds, pulses and beans - add vitamin C foods (berries, citrus fruit, tomatoes, peppers etc) or a supplement.

Good fats for cell membrane repair and anti-inflammatory - oily fish, olive oil, coconut oil, avocados, nuts and seeds.

Protein rich foods - building blocks: meat, fish, poultry, tofu, beans, lentils, full fat yoghurt & cheese, eggs, nuts, seeds, alfalfa.

Zinc, skin and tissue healing: Oysters, red meat, poultry, baked beans, chickpeas, cashews, almonds, tofu, pork, seeds, lentils, yoghurt, oatmeal and mushrooms.

4. Breastfeeding

Women should be aware that after a caesarean section, it may take longer for the milk to come in and for the baby's instincts to "wake up". Engage a lactation consultant at the earliest need.

5. The baby

Microbiome introduction - either a swab (called seeding) or otherwise loads of skin-to-skin and breastfeeding.

- Imitate the womb and have the baby with the mother as soon as possible. Skin-to-skin with the partner until then.
- Wait with the first bath until the umbilical cord is off. Limit handling of the baby by non-family members.

TIPS : *Place a maternity pad (with the sticky side out) over your wound to reduce friction between the wound and clothing/bedding. Have a soft pillow or cuddly toy at hand to hold against your wound as counter pressure when laughing, sneezing or coughing.*

Contractions

CONTRACTIONS DURING LABOUR THIN out and open the cervix, the "exit" of the womb.

During labour and birth contractions accomplish two things: (1) they cause the cervix to thin and dilate (open); and (2) they help push the baby down into the birth canal.

The hormone oxytocin, which plays a role in love, bonding, reduction of stress, breastfeeding and healing is also responsible for regulating labour contractions. Oxytocin receptors on the uterus slowly increase towards the end of pregnancy and when the pituitary gland releases oxytocin, which is most likely triggered by the baby) these receptors enable the uterus to begin contracting.

Contractions start in the top of the uterus (fundus) and 'wave' downwards. The cervix must be ready (ripe) before it will respond to contractions by opening (dilating). Initially contractions can be irregular in length, strength and time.

To begin, the mildness of and the long pauses between contractions facilitate the mother's ability to do what is needed to hunker down and move into established labour. She may need to get home, alert her partner, organise her other children, call her midwife and birth companions, travel to a birth centre or hospital, etc.

Due to the fine balance of hormones during labour and birth the contractions can be inhibited at this early stage in response to stress (danger) in the same way as other mammals would.

It can take many hours or even days for this early labour phase to tip over into established labour.

Contraction pattern and strength

Generally contractions are measured according to how often they occur in a 10 minute period although each woman's contraction pattern is unique and there are ample women who manage to birth their babies with diverse contraction patterns.

During a contraction the placental circulation is reduced (more so if the membranes have ruptured), slightly decreasing the oxygen supply to the baby. This is why there are breaks in between contractions – to allow the baby to rebalance their oxygen levels before the next contraction with the added bonus that the mother also has breaks in which her body is able to produce beta-endorphins as a crucial part of the labour process.

Most women will experience a tightening and hardening of their uterus called Braxton-Hicks contractions which increase in regularity and strength in the last two to three weeks of their pregnancy. When labour contractions begin, they will feel more like menstrual cramping and as labour progresses they slowly build becoming more intense and closer together.

Every labour is different and each woman will experience her contractions differently but as labour progresses the contractions will become longer, - at least forty-five to seventy-five seconds each - stronger and progressively more frequent, going from one contraction every ten to fifteen minutes to one every five minutes and eventually to one every two to three minutes. As the dilation nears ten centimetres the contractions could be as frequent as one every minute.

Contractions tend to come in waves, they have a beginning, a peak and an ebbing away. Having said that, contractions could begin suddenly and could already be only three minutes apart OR they can be very irregular and very strong from the start.

A question commonly asked in my practice is, *"How will I know that the contractions have started?"* The best bet is that if you are in doubt then they probably aren't labour contractions, but as I have said before, each labour is different and each woman will experience her labour contractions differently.

Changing your activity at that moment can sometimes help to clarify things. If you are resting; take a walk, if you are walking; go home and rest. If what you believe (conceive) to be contractions stop with this change, then it is not yet "time".

Promoting effective contractions

The birth team will need to concentrate on creating an environment that supports oxytocin release to ensure strong, regular contractions.

Go to the chapter about the Hormones of Labour and Birth -> #chapter=qg5NUd9REy4Hv86A

Continuity of Care

The term "continuity of care" means having the same midwife or doctor throughout pregnancy, childbirth and postpartum. Specifically, continuous support during labour from the same maternity caregiver has been associated with a positive childbirth experience. This is referred to as "relational continuity" or "personal continuity" which supports trust and familiarity between care provider and the client / patient. Other dimensions of continuity of care are "information continuity" in which the care provider uses and exchanges information on past events to deliver care that is appropriate to the patient's current circumstances and "management continuity" in which the care providers connect their care in a coherent way.

The Benefits of Continuity of Care

- More chance of spontaneous vaginal birth
- Have a more positive experience of labour and birth

- Be satisfied with her maternity care
- Successfully breastfeed her baby
- Cost the health system less
- Less likely to have regional analgesia
- Better health outcomes

In summary

Care from a known midwife, or the same doctor, enables women to develop a relationship with their care providers. Women who have the same care provider caring for them during pregnancy, labour, birth and post birth have the opportunity to build a trusting relationship which increases their confidence.

Being a recipient of continuity of care and becoming comfortable with someone, building a relationship with them which grows and deepens over time, enables trust to develop and women begin to share their deeper anxieties and insecurities as well as enjoying the more positive aspects of growing knowledge and confidence through a supported journey of discovery.

> *Midwives also benefit from the continuity of care model. For a midwife, getting to know the woman, and developing a trusting relationship with her during her pregnancy, is the best way for her to support the woman to have a safe, positive and empowering birth experience, whilst maintain-*

ing and strengthening clinical expertise across all areas of maternity care.

Delayed (Optimal) Cord Clamping

THE UMBILICAL CORD LINKS your placenta to the baby. After your baby has been born, the umbilical cord continues to pulsate because it is transferring much needed blood, oxygen, and stem cells to your baby while they adjust to being outside the womb.

It *used to be* common practice to cut the umbilical cord straight after the baby was born. Now, according to guidelines, it is normal practice to wait until the cord has stopped pulsating and becomes white before cutting the cord. The midwife or doctor are able to feel when this happens by just touching the cord and can take anything from 1 minute to 20 minutes -> https://apps.who.int/iris/bitstream/handle/10665/148793/9789241508209_eng.pdf;jsessionid=493B30184E55C131B69D7875EF9ADF2B?sequence=1

By delaying the clamping of the cord, more essential blood travels from the cord and placenta to the baby.

Why is delayed (or optimal) cord clamping recommended?

The benefits of delayed cord clamping include:

- Increased iron levels in the baby even up until they are 4 months old, which helps with growth and both physical and emotional development.

- Increased amount of stem cells, which helps with a baby's growth and helps with their immune system.

- Studies have shown that neurodevelopment of the baby is enhanced when the cord clamping is delayed.

- There is research that suggests that delayed cord clamping can improve the health of term and preterm babies ->

https://www.acog.org/clinical/clinical-guidance/committee-opinion/articles/2020/12/delayed-umbilical-cord-clamping-after-birth

Delayed cord clamping during a C-section

This same study above, also looked at delaying cord clamping by 30 seconds during a cesarean section showed that these babies have higher iron reserves at 4 months than those who had their cords clamped immediately.

Lotus Birth

Some parents choose to leave their baby attached to the placenta until the umbilical cord falls off naturally (usually between three to seven days after birth, depending on humidity).

Dilation

As labour nears, the cervix may start to thin (efface) and open (dilate). Dilation is measured in centimetres. Fully dilated means that the cervix has dilated to around 10 centimetres and that your baby is able to move into the birth canal and is ready to be pushed out once you get the urge to push.

How fast the cervix effaces and dilates varies for each woman. In some women, the cervix may start to efface and dilate slowly in the last weeks of pregnancy but it is usual for first-time mothers' to begin dilating once labour starts.

Dilation is determined by a care provider doing a vaginal examination. They insert two fingers into the vagina to reach the cervix in order to feel the condition and position of the cervix.

NOTE: Although dilation of the cervix is essential for the progression of labour, it is just one part of the complex and multidimensional birth process. What the cervix is doing at the moment of a vaginal examination does not indicate what the cervix is going to do in the future. Therefore, the findings cannot always effectively inform decisions made about the progression of labour.

Some midwives and doctors like to check the condition, position, effacement and possible dilation at the end of pregnancy before labour begins. The result of what is felt is referred to as a Bishops score. A Bishops score is UNABLE to predict when labour might begin and should not be used as such. It is unreliable and inaccurate. The only function of a Bishops score is to assess whether a cervix is ready for certain kinds of induction.

ENGAGEMENT OF THE BABY'S HEAD

From about 33 weeks onward of your pregnancy, you may experience your baby moving lower down into your pelvis. This process is known as "engagement" or "lightening" and simply means that the leading part of the baby has entered into the pelvic brim. This helps to position the baby in preparation for the birth when it comes.

Your care provider will usually record when this has occurred during one of your antenatal checks. Women often experience "engaging contractions" when the baby engages. These can be quite painful and are often experienced as a false start to labour.

Many women report feeling more physically at ease following the head engaging. You may feel it is easier to breath, sleep and you may have less heartburn or indigestion. On the other hand the engaged head may lead to increased pressure on your bladder and you may feel a sensation of fullness and pressure between your legs.

> *Additional information: In first pregnancies, the baby's head tends to engage during the last month. However in subsequent pregnancies it is not unusual for the head to only engage with the onset of labour.*

EATING & DRINKING DURING LABOUR

IT IS ESSENTIAL THAT you eat and drink when you can during labour and birth in order to sustain the process. It's usually best to be guided by what you *feel* like eating while you are in early labour. Once you're in strong, full blown labour, you will probably not want to eat much at all, just make sure you are hydrating.

A snack every hour in the early stages can go a long way to storing up energy for the work ahead.

Examples of foods to eat and drink in early labour

- Small baked potato topped with some cream cheeseAvocado on toast

- Peanut butter sandwichesPasta with a light sauce

- Rice with soy sauce

- Hummus

HOLISTIC CHILDBIRTH MANUAL

- A bowl of cereal
- Yoghurt
- Dried fruit
- Fresh fruit
- Nuts
- Smoothie
- Celery & carrot sticksEnergy barsRaisinsRice cakes/crackers
- Energy balls
- Dates
- Jelly
- Sorbet ice lolliesFrozen grapes or berries
- Chicken soup – it is sometimes nice to just drink the clear bouillon of chicken soup and to save the more hearty part for after the birth
- Vegetable soup
- Tea
- Hot Chocolate

NOTE: Foods high in sugar may give you that quick energy boost at the end when you need to regroup for pushing but earlier in labour they may leave you

feeling tired and nauseous once the energy peak you get from sugar is over.

Stay hydrated throughout

Labour is thirsty work and sometimes it can be a challenge to stay hydrated. Add maple syrup or honey (one teaspoon per 500ml) and bicarbonate of soda (1/4 teaspoon per 500ml) to help you avoid becoming dehydrated. Dehydration will cause a lactic build up in your muscles; specifically the uterine muscles which are working hard during labour, and lactic build up will make the contractions sharper and more painful.

Episiotomy

An episiotomy was once routinely practiced during childbirth. It is a surgical cut made in the muscular area between the vagina and the anus (the perineum) with the intention to enlarge the vaginal opening to either avoid tearing or to speed up the birth. The incision needs extensive suturing to close it up.

Routine episiotomies are no longer recommended. has proven that they do not prevent tearing, they do not always aid in the birth being quicker, they take longer to heal and have more complications than a spontaneous vaginal tear and they have more long term side effects. Also, women who have episiotomies tend to lose more blood at the time of birth, have more pain during recovery, and have to wait longer before having sex without discomfort. Sometimes an episiotomy damages the anal sphincter increasing the risk of anal incontinence, which means trouble controlling bowel movements and gas.

FACT: Studies show that midwives do far fewer episiotomies than obstetricians.

Although there is no consensus on how frequently the procedure should be used, a leading hospital safety group recommends that episiotomies should occur in no more than 5% of vaginal births. Prenatal appointments are a good time to ask your healthcare provider about how often they make the cuts and for what reasons? "You want to hear: I rarely cut episiotomies," It should be a shared decision-making conversation between you and your healthcare professional.

Ways to help avoid an episiotomy

There are alternatives to the risk of tearing during the birth such as applying warm compresses to the perineum during the pushing stage to help the tissue become softer and more pliable.

A technique called perineal massage helps the tissue relax and become more flexible and resistant to tearing. A showed that women who hadn't previously given birth who started perineal massage at 34 weeks of pregnancy had 10% reduced risk of a tear requiring sutures than women who didn't practice perineal massage.

During labour, use strategies and techniques that can help increase your chance of an uncomplicated birth, such as continuous labour support from a midwife or a doula.

Most episiotomies are carried out when a doctor needs to use instruments (like a vacuum or forceps) to help your baby to be born. You'll be more likely to need this kind of intervention if you have an epidural, so you may prefer pain management techniques such as the TENS or gas and air as pain relief options.

Try to stay in an upright position when pushing to allow gravity to help. Choosing a different position from lying on your back, such as kneeling on all fours, squatting, standing or lying on your side, can help you give birth without the need for an episiotomy.

Foetal Monitoring in Labour

CARE PROVIDERS LISTEN TO the baby's heart during labour as part of their labour assessment. There are two methods of listening, *intermittent auscultation* (IA) and *continuous electronic monitoring* (CEFM) via a cardiotocograph machine (CTG).

Intermittent auscultation (IA)

Some midwives will use a Pinnard. It is a trumpet-shaped wooden instrument through which the midwife can hear the baby's heart sounds directly. Some may use a fetoscope (similar to a stethoscope) but most midwives will use a doppler to intermittently listen to the baby's heart rate during labour. The Doppler uses short pulses of ultrasound waves to detect movement and turns those movements into sound.

> If you are birthing with a midwife (no matter the setting) and you are at

low-risk then you have the right to request intermittent auscultation because the The American Congress of Obstetrics and Gynecologists does not endorse CEFM for low-risk pregnancies.

Continuous electronic monitoring (CEFM)

Most clinicians working in hospital settings will want to continually trace the baby's heart rate during labour with CEFM where a continuous CTG **produces a paper recording of the baby's heart rate and the mother's labour contractions**. shows that low-risk mothers do not need CEFM as it restricts freedom of maternal movement, can create stress in the mother and has not shown to improve infant outcomes.

HORMONES OF LABOUR AND BIRTH

THE KEY HORMONES OF labour and birth

Oxytocin: love, bonding, reduction of stress, healing, uterine contractions, breastfeeding.

Beta-endorphins: pain relief, activation of reward centres in the brain, altered state of consciousness – 'transcendence'.

Epinephrine and Norepinephrine also known as adrenaline and noradrenaline: stress hormones (shorter-term activation). "Flight or fight "trigger.

Prolactin: mothering hormone, lactation.

FACT: It is valuable for birthing women to understand that the hormones during labour will modify their brain. Making it possible for them to imagine that the baby is going to be born.

The cocktail of hormones, which are triggered at childbirth are common to all mammals and originate deep in the mammalian brain. For birth to proceed optimally, this part of the brain must take precedence over the neocortex, also known as our rational (thinking) brain. Dim lighting, little conversation, reassurance, gentle support and no expectations or rationality from you as the labouring woman can help achieve this. You will then intuitively choose the movements, sounds, breathing and positions that will help you to birth your baby most efficiently. This is your genetic and hormonal blueprint, which you can access only if your rational brain is relegated to the background.

A closer look at Oxytocin

Oxytocin reduces stress by centrally activating the parasympathetic nervous system, which promotes calm, connection, healing and growth. It reduces fear, stress, and stress hormones plus it increases sociability by reducing activity in the sympathetic nervous system.

Oxytocin causes your uterine (womb) muscles to contract, which in turn causes your cervix to become thin and dilate (open.) During labour your body continues to produce oxytocin to facilitate the birthing process, it also ensures the release of your placenta, helps reduce blood loss after birth and it is released to stimulate the let-down response in breastfeeding.

Oxytocin release during labour is inhibited (suppressed) by the production of adrenaline and noradrenaline (epinephrine and norepinephrine) which in turn are triggered by stress, fear, loud noises, strangers coming into your labour room/space, unfamiliar or hostile birth environments, interruptions and distractions, interventions (such as vaginal exams) lack of privacy and acute embarrassment.

> ***On the question of "privacy" and labour, Michel Odent, a renowned obstetrician states; "The right place to give birth would be the right place to make love" (Odent, 1982.)***

Oxytocin also helps us in our emotional and physical transition to motherhood. Oxytocin encourages us to "forget ourselves", either through altruism — service to others — or through feelings of love.

Oxytocin also causes the perfect "warm place" for the newborn through vasodilation of mothers' blood circulation to her chest - this literally makes her chest the warmest place for the baby to be.

A closer look at Adrenaline

Adrenaline is a hormone that has a profound effect, both negative and positive on labour and birth.

The negative effect of adrenaline during labour

When the natural flow of your labour is disturbed, the body takes instinctive, evasive action to ensure survival and protection by "stopping" the labour in order to create time and the possibility of finding a safe space for you and your unborn baby.

This survival mechanism produces adrenaline, the "flight or fight" hormone. Producing adrenaline is an automatic response in any frightening or threatening situation. The release of adrenaline inhibits the release of oxytocin (the hormone needed to stimulate contractions), which can stop contractions or slow down the labour process.

What a birthing partner can do if an overproduction of adrenaline is slowing the birth process.

Firstly a birth partner needs to identify the source of fear or disturbance and try to remove it.

Where possible one or more of the following panic control measures can be introduced:

- Provide privacy.

- Reassurance, massage, Bach rescue remedy, a warm shower or bath, acupressure, rhythmic movements and humming.

- Avoid unnecessary discussions and avoid asking the birthing mother too many questions.

- Change the environment but only if this is the threat because a move can also cause the release of adrenaline.

- Dim the lights and aim to provide warmth and quiet.

- Reduce birth attendants, beginning with unnecessary staff or family members.

- Remove anyone who is showing signs of anxiety.

- Be aware that the "danger" which the birthing mother experienced can come in many nuances.

Allow at least an hour for the adrenaline levels to decrease and for endorphins and oxytocin to reappear once the situation has been addressed.

The positive effect of adrenaline during the pushing phase of labour Adrenaline is essential in a normal birth during your final contractions just before the birth of your baby. The presence of adrenaline can be physically seen in the way you gain energy, become more focused and obtain new strength and alertness at this time. The baby also gets a burst of foetal adrenaline; this allows it to be born alert with wide-open eyes and dilated pupils, which encourages bonding.

Thanks to the hormones, the scene is set for a dependent baby who wants and needs love and protection, born to a mother who is primed to love strongly and protectively.

Beta-endorphins

Beta-endorphins give analgesic and adaptive responses to stress and pain. They activate brain reward and pleasure centres, motivating and rewarding reproductive and social behaviours, and support immune function, physical activity, and psychological well-being.

Beta-endorphins offer a number of benefits for you during labour:

- They are natural painkillers

- They create a sense of wellbeing and promote positive feelings

- They are an important link in mother-baby attachment; creating a positive emotional climate for the first meeting with the baby

- Create an altered state of consciousness that supports the birthing woman to deal with stress and pain

- The endorphins work as painkillers for the baby during labour and help with the stress of postpartum transition

You are able to influence how effectively your body is able to produce endorphins during labour by being as relaxed and calm as possible **during the PAUSES between contractions** - this is when the endorphins are produced. Being tense and distracted between contractions inhibits the production of this natural pain relief.

Certain techniques such as massage, gentle touch, warmth and acupressure help to increase the amount of endorphins a body makes.

> *These powerful pain relieving endorphins are specifically produced during the PAUSES between contractions. Finding ways to be calm and relaxed BETWEEN contractions is the best way to tap into these beneficial hormones.*

Prolactin

Prolactin is entwined with oxytocin. It stimulates the parasympathetic nervous system, it reduces anxiety.

When prolactin is combined with oxytocin, as it is soon after birth and during breastfeeding, it encourages a relaxed and selfless devotion to the baby that contributes to a mother's satisfaction and her baby's physical and emotional health.

INDUCTION OF LABOUR

INDUCTION OF LABOUR IS and should only be carried out when there is a medical complication that threatens either the health of the mother and/or her baby. There are some medical complications that require labour to be induced such as pre-eclampsia, poor growth of the baby, an infection, when there's not enough amniotic fluid surrounding the baby etc.

Another reason is having pre-labour rupture of membranes with no contractions to follow - each country's care provider and facility has its own decided time limit given for contractions to start after the rupture of membranes.

The most common reason for induction is a prolonged pregnancy.

All Induction carries risks and the choice to induce for prolonged pregnancy should be made only once there is an understanding of all the options and associated risks of not being induced versus being induced. Risk is a very personal concept and different women will consider different risks to be significant to them once they have received individualized information. Only with this information are they able to choose the option with the risks they are most willing to take.

The idea of a prolonged pregnancy assumes that all women are pregnant for exactly the same amount of time. However, it seems that genetic differences may influence what is a 'normal' gestation time for a particular woman. Meaning that if the women in your family gestate for 42 weeks so might you.

Other factors are a possible miscalculation of the due date, diet and lifestyle and most first time mothers tend to gestate a little longer.

Possible risks in waiting for spontaneous labour

Aging placenta

There is a misconceived belief that the placenta has a 'best used before' date and that it starts to deteriorate after 40 weeks. There is evidence that the structure and biochemistry of the placenta changes as pregnancy develops to adapt to meet the changing needs of the baby however there is no logical reason for believing that the placenta, which is a foetal organ, should age while the other foetal organs do not. Tests of placental function show no changes in post-dates pregnancies.

Big baby

Women have concerns that the baby will grow too big and therefore be difficult to birth. There is evidence that babies continue to grow bigger the longer they gestate, and this contradicts the above theory about the aging placenta. *If the placenta stops functioning, how does the baby continue to grow so well?* Big babies are pretty good at finding their way out of their mothers expandable pelvis. The research about complications relating to big babies suggests that it is the interventions carried out when a baby is assumed to be big rather than the actual size of the baby.

Risk associated with Induction

It can be difficult to untangle and isolate the risks involved with induction because usually more than one risk factor is occurring at once (e.g., synthetic oxytocin, CTG, epidural). In addition, there are differences in outcomes and risks between women who have previously laboured, and women having their first baby. It is important for women to consider their own individual factors and how these alter their individual risk profile.

Induction of labour is known to cause iatrogenic (medically caused) prematurity.

Most labours start spontaneously, given time. This allows for your body to move through each part of labour as it builds up. In this way your body is able to release endorphins so that both you and your baby are able to cope with the ever- increasing intensity of the contractions. With medical induction this natural succession is by-passed.

It has been clearly shown that one or a combination of the methods used to induce labour can lead to foetal distress and for this reason, once an induction is set in motion, the baby needs to be be carefully monitored which restricts a woman's freedom to move around, which makes it harder for her to cope with the intensity of induced labour.

When labour is induced using medication, it may take longer, contractions tend to be more painful and babies tend to end up in positions that make it harder for them to move through the pelvis and down the birth canal.

With the baby being in a less favourable position and because pain relief is needed, the natural urge to push is not felt, resulting in more assisted deliveries with either forceps or vacuum extraction.

The use of prolonged synthetic oxytocin increases the risk of postpartum bleeding.

Increased Risk of C-Section because if one method doesn't kick-start contractions, then more interventions are needed in the management of the labour resulting in a cascade of interventions which increases the possibility of a C-section. A C-section is also more likely if the baby is in a less favourable position for being born vaginally. Foetal distress is a common reason during an induction for doing a C-section.

Medically induced labour will need managing; unlike physiological labour and birth.

Methods of induction

Membrane stretch-and-sweep

Membrane sweeping involves a care provider placing a finger (or two) just inside your cervix and making a circular, sweeping movement to separate the membranes from the inner part of the cervix. Your membranes can only be swept once your cervix opens enough for your care provider to insert a finger.

Induction is being 'offered' more frequently, and a stretch and sweep is seen by many as an attempt to avoid hospital induction of labour.

A stretch and sweep cannot be done if your membranes have ruptured because of the increased risk of infection.

Risks of a stretch and sweep

The risks and downsides of a stretch and sweep include discomfort and irregular contractions, which may interfere with your ability to rest and sleep in the last few days of pregnancy and there is a chance it won't get labour started.

A vaginal examination always carries a risk of infection.

There is a risk of rupturing the membranes. If this happens, it means that, because there is now a risk of infection, hospital induction will be offered if you do not go into labour within a certain time.

Many women find vaginal examinations embarrassing and/or uncomfortable.

Prostaglandins

Prostaglandin tablets or gel are given to "prime" the cervix to get the cervix shorter and softer and to possibly induce uterine contractions. If prostaglandins do not induce contractions then it is a way to move onto the next stage of induction which would be to either rupture membranes or begin with medical oxytocin. If your membranes have not yet ruptured then prostaglandins are often the recommended method of induction.

Prostaglandins are usually given as a capsule or gel that is inserted into the vagina every six to eight hours. More than one dose is often needed to induce labour.

Risks of using prostaglandins

Prostaglandins may lead to hyper stimulation resulting in foetal distress and a C-section.

Most women will not go into labour with prostaglandins and will require further induction methods.

Foley catheter (Foleys balloon)

This method can only be done if your membranes have not ruptured. A catheter with a very small un-inflated balloon at the end is inserted up into your cervix, between your inner cervix and your baby's head. The balloon is then inflated with a saline solution so that it puts pressure on your cervix from the inside, stimulating the release of prostaglandins. This causes the cervix to soften and open (dilate) and typically around 3 to 5cm dilated, the balloon falls out and the catheter is removed.

The goal of this method is to cause your cervix to mechanically open. Sometimes this will start labour spontaneously or it may simply make your cervix more favourable for other methods of induction like rupturing your membranes (amniotomy) or the use of synthetic oxytocin.

Risks of a Foley catheter

There is an increased risk of infection and it is often said to be uncomfortable and is sometimes experienced as painful.

Rupturing the membranes (amniotomy)

In some countries care providers will manually break your amniotic bag of water to attempt to induce labour. This is also known as an amniotomy.

An amniotomy is done by inserting an amnihook (a long implement that looks like a large crochet hook), and snagging the amniotic membranes. By creating this tear in the bag, the amniotic fluid will begin to leak out.

The actual breaking of the bag of water shouldn't be any more painful than any other vaginal examination. Sometimes the rupturing of the membranes triggers contractions.

If you were having contractions before your water was surgically ruptured, this is called augmenting labour and not inducing labour.

Risks associated with rupturing the membranes:

- Failure of labour to start
- Having to move onto using medical oxytocin
- Foetal distress
- Increase in foetal mal-position
- Incrcased risk of a C-section

- Increased risk of infection
- Increased pain experience of labour contractions

Medical oxytocin IV

Oxytocin (also known as Syntocinon or Pitocin) is a drug that is used to stimulate the uterus to contract. It is given via an IV into your bloodstream. The use of medical oxytocin requires continuous monitoring of the baby's heart rate for the duration of your labour as use of this drug may affect the length and intensity of the contractions which may cause foetal distress. The continuous monitoring and being attached to a drip will affect your ability to move around during your labour

If your membranes have not ruptured, then an amniotomy will be recommended in order to apply something called a foetal scalp electrode which is attached to the baby's head in order to continuously monitor the baby.

Because medical oxytocin does not have the same pain relieving effects of the body's own oxytocin, it is common for women to need an epidural to help them to cope with labour pain.

It is known that oxytocin can overstimulate the uterus and if this happens you could be asked to lie on your left hand side and the drip will be turned down or off to lessen the contractions. Sometimes another drug will be given to counteract the oxytocin and lessen the contractions.

It is then a fine balance of stimulating contractions in order to have labour progression and not to cause foetal distress.

INVITING LABOUR NATURALLY

Although we are not entirely sure, studies show that the initiation of labour is likely caused by the baby secreting a substance (surfactant protein and platelet-activating factor) into the amniotic fluid as their lungs mature. This results in an inflammatory response in the mother's uterus that initiates labour. We have not found one definitive way to "make" this happen because all babies' lungs mature at different times generally within the five week period (37 - 42 weeks gestation). What we do know is that a mother with nervous system dis-regulation which results in a state of chronic stress, subliminal messages her body (via the sympathetic nervous system) and her baby that it is not safe for labour to begin.

There are a variation of therapies, techniques and measures that can be tried to help a woman's body to go into labour. There is no proof (other than in the pudding) that these things work for everyone or all the time. What is clear is that it helps for women to not feel entirely helpless and it gives them incentive to not choose for induction without at least trying something less invasive.

In situations where we know that stress is getting in the way we can endeavour to help the mother to move more into her parasympathetic nervous system and out of her sympathetic nervous system.

Parasympathetic Nervous System

Hormones of birth create behaviours and thoughts but only function properly if the body is predominantly in the parasympathetic nervous system, also known as our Rest and Digest state. It slows anxiety and overthinking.

Sympathetic nervous system

The sympathetic nervous system Is ruled by the thinking brain (neocortex). It keeps us in our state of "doing" and is the state of fight or flight.

Hacking the Parasympathetic Nervous System via the Vagus Nerve

The vagus nerve is a long meandering bundle of motor and sensory fibres that links the brain stem to the salivary glands, heart, lungs, diaphragm, gut, ovaries and uterus.

The vagus nerve is the key to the parasympathetic nervous system and when stimulated:

- It activates the parasympathetic system and acts to counterbalance the fight or flight system.

- It is involved with oxytocin release.

- It triggers intuition.

- It enhances feelings of calm and safety.

Stimulating the Vagus Nerve

Certain actions will tap into the vagus nerve, which in turn, switches our body into the parasympathetic nervous system, which sends a message to our body to say "I am safe". Once the body shifts into this place of feeling safe, it can then more easily move into labour.

- Deep/slow soft-belly breathing humming on the out breath

- Physiological Sighing

- Humming

- Filling the mouth with saliva and submerging your tongue to trigger a hyper-relaxing vagal response - if the mouth feels dry then take a small sip of cold water and hold it in your mouth to submerge your tongue

- Meditation

- Self-hypnosis

Other ways of inviting labour to begin

A combination of two or more of the following techniques may help you move into labour if you have passed your due date; preferably already 41 weeks.

These techniques focus on the mother's body and mind and will have no influence over the baby actually being "ready" to be born. BUT, imagine the baby is ready but the mother's state of mind or lack of balance is a little out-of-whack then it may be just the trigger she needs.

Acupuncture

Acupuncture for induction involves the insertion of very fine needles into specific points of the body to encourage the body to take that last step towards going into labour. Acupuncture to induce an over- due labour will generally be started around forty-one weeks and three days and you may need two to three sessions on consecutive days. Acupuncture can help to relax you and get your mind off the waiting, which can be just the trigger your body needs to go into labour. Acupuncture will not induce labour if both your body and the baby are not ready for labour.

Nipple stimulation

Stimulating your nipples by rolling them or using a breastmilk pump may help increase the levels of oxytocin. The usual recommendation is fifteen minutes of continual stimulation on each nipple each hour for several hours. If your contractions start, continue until they are regular and then stop the stimulation.

Sex

Sex as means of getting labour started is thought to work in four ways: firstly the physical movement may help to stimulate the uterus into action; secondly, sex can trigger the release of oxytocin, thirdly, if you orgasm the orgasmic contractions may stimulate labour contractions and thirdly, semen contains high concentrations of prostaglandins which help to ripen (soften) your cervix. Sex is safe as long as your membranes have not ruptured.

Evening Primrose Oil

Evening Primrose Oil (EPO) is commonly used by midwives to help ripen the cervix in the last few weeks of pregnancy. One 500mg capsule is taken daily and two gel capsules (each 500mg) are inserted vaginally and pushed up against the cervix before bedtime.Use clean fingers and make sure the capsules are also clean. Inserting anything into the vagina during pregnancy increases the risk of infection.

Reflexology

Reflexology can both stimulate and relax. It is used worldwide as part of natural induction.

Homeopathy

A homeopath will be able to advise which remedy or remedies you may need to help get labour started.

Herbs

A herbalist will be able to advise which herbs you could try to help get labour started.

Walking

Walking (uphill or up and down stairs) might help to trigger labour. The explanation as to how, is that the pressure of your baby's head on the cervix stimulates the release of oxytocin. Also, just being upright gets the forces of gravity working for you, encouraging the baby to move down onto the cervix. Take a brisk walk every evening before bedtime, but don't wear yourself out, labour can be exhausting and you don't want to use up all your energy before you've begun.

Castor oil

Using castor oil is really the last resort and should only be used in agreement with a care provider or health practitioner. It acts as a powerful laxative stimulating the intestine which in turn stimulates the uterus. Castor oil also contains prostaglandins; the hormones needed to soften and prepare the cervix.

Castor oil cocktail ingredients: please note that the recipe for the castor oil cocktail is very specific and needs to be accurately followed:

300ml of thick (not clear) juice like apricot or mango.2 50ml of sparkling water

2 tablespoons of castor oil2 tablespoons of lemon verbena oil2 tablespoons of almond or peanut butter

Place the ingredients in a jar that has a lid and shake to mix - be careful when opening due to the effervescence of the sparkling water. Drink the entire decoction then take a hot shower and lie down on your left side.

Nausea will most likely be the immediate effect of castor oil, ensuring to keep it down. The wanted effect should be felt within 4 hours. This is a bad case of diarrhoea. Ensure you are close to a toilet and be mindful of hygiene; diarrhoea can be a messy business.

Extreme diarrhoea can lead to dehydration, be sure to stay well hydrated to compensate for the loss of liquid.

Labour

I N *OBSTETRICALLY DEFINED* LANGUAGE, and pertaining to first births, labour is divided into three distinct stages and phases within the stages:

- **First stage** involves regular, coordinated uterine contractions accompanied by cervical dilatation. The **first stage** has **three phases: latent, active** and **transition.**

- **Second stage** begins when the cervix is fully dilated and ends when the baby is born.

- **Third stage** is the delivery of the placenta and membranes and ends with the control of bleeding'

Each labour unfolds differently

Every woman's labour is different and how your body births will depend on whether it is your first or 5th baby, how the baby is positioned in your pelvis, surrounding circumstances, how you feel and so forth. There is not one pattern of labour that fits all.

In this chapter, I will attempt to highlight the important factors to help you understand the biology of labour and birth a little better. This in turn may help you to labour more efficiently or at least give you a road map to guide you through your labour, however it goes.

> *Labour and birth is not just about "getting the baby out" it is about the entire (necessary) process that leads to you and your baby finally meeting.*

❖

How physiological, spontaneous, labour may unfold *without* specifically focussing on the obstetrically defined stages and phases.

IN THE BEGINNING

What can we observe on the outside

In early labour the contractions are generally without a real pattern. They can be short - 40 seconds or less - and far apart - every 20 mins or more.

Contractions are felt in the lower abdomen and don't radiate out much.

You may have mucous or bloody show.

There may be an emptying of bowels.

Contractions are likely to slow or stop in response to a journey to hospital or other stressful/distracting situations.

What's happening internally

The cervix ripens and may efface.

The cervix dilates anything from 1 to 3 centimetres - only known if the care provider is doing vaginal examinations.

Your (possible) behaviour

You are able to have your open between and during contractions.

You are able to hold a conversation and answer questions and/or to engage with external activities e.g., using your phone to time contractions.

You might feel excitement, anxiety and uncertainty.

You may be keen to get settled into your chosen birth space.

You are able to easily walk upright between contractions.

What you may need

A walk, watch a movie or a sleep - whichever is appropriate.

Healthy light foods/snacks.

Hydration.

Time to wind down and arrange logistics - getting the "nest" ready.

WHEN THINGS START BECOMING MORE INTENSE

What can we observe on the outside

The contractions become more intense, they become more regular, longer and closer together.

Contractions can be felt in the entire belly, the lower back, radiating through the buttocks and down the thighs.

Your membranes might rupture.

Labour is now established.

What's happening internally

Your cervix is dilating from 4/6 cm until 7/8 cm - only known if the care provider is doing vaginal examinations.

Your baby is moving down further into the pelvis.

Your (possible) behaviour

You begin to turn more inward, letting go of your usual state of consciousness and your connection to the external world - you are generally non-communicative.

You are focused on getting through each contraction.

You are more serious.

You may mention that you feel tired - you may be tired from working hard but this could also be a sign of good levels of endorphins.

You are no longer able to be in a normal upright posture - you may need to be on hands and knees, lying on your side, hanging from or onto something, bending forward and leaning etc.

What you may need

You will be more likely to need and ask for support and positive encouragement.

You may try techniques you learnt in pregnancy like acupressure, massage, TENS machine, counter pressure, breathing techniques, hypnobirthing etc. Via a QR code in the bonus materials you can download a PDF with details about using acupressure and counter pressure during labour and birth.

Hydration - you will be thirsty.

You will want to get into a birth pool or a shower depending what you have chosen for.

Regular change of position.

Rhythmic movement or sounds.

THE LAST SPRINT (before pushing)

What can we observe on the outside

The dilation of the last few centimetres sometimes begins with a lull in the contractions. We call this a rest and be thankful moment. Not all women experience this.

The contractions that open the very last centimetre's become very intense, they may have multiple peaks and come very close together - one a minute.

They can last sixty to ninety seconds.

Your movements and sounds will be instinctive and rhythmical.

Your inhibitions reduce.

Your membranes might rupture - if they haven't already.

What's happening internally

The cervix dilates the final centimetres

The baby begins to move further down, rotating around and moving down through the pelvis.

Your (possible) behaviour

You will likely need to vocalise during contractions – often the same noise with each one.

You may have a dry mouth and might suddenly be very thirsty.

You may feel as if you have tunnel vision.

You could find it difficult to express your needs.

You will seem to be sensitive to everything - too hot, too cold, touch me, no don't touch me...

You may express feelings of fear and being overwhelmed.

You may feel convinced that you cannot do this anymore and have irrational requests like asking for the pain relief you (definitely) didn't want.

You may be nauseous and need to vomit.

You may be shaking and trembling.

You could start to make sounds of grunting or feel a catch in your breath.

What you may need

To cover your eyes - keep out any light.

Heating pads for your lower back.

Acupressure – via a QR code in the bonus materials you can download a PDF with details about using acupressure during labour and birth.

Not being touched or needing to be touched.

PUSHING THE BABY OUT

What can we observe on the outside

There may be a lull in contractions as the uterus 'reorganises' itself around the baby as it moves down.

You may begin to have the spontaneous urge to bear down - which may feel to you as if you need to poop; you will most likely voice this. It may take a while for you to recognise that you are feeling the urge to push rather than a bowel movement urge.

You may see a little amount of poop at this stage. It is never very much and is literally being squeezed out like the last bit of toothpaste in a tube.

The contractions space out and become "expulsive" - a more obvious downward wave as the uterus helps to move the baby down and out.

Your noises and behaviour will change.

Your (possible) behaviour

You may reach up or forward and arch your back.

You become more awake and aware.

You may feel the need to be upright so that gravity can help the baby to descend.

BIRTH OF THE PLACENTA

Contractions continue after the baby is born. They cause the placenta to detach & to be pushed out of the uterus.

Less intense contractions, called after pains, will then begin to shrink the uterus back to its original size.

General, additional information around labour and birth

Although the length of labour varies considerably, women experiencing their first full-term birth generally have the longest labours. Once labour has established a strong pattern about half will exceed twelve hours, and two in ten labours will last longer than twenty-four hours. Subsequent labours tend to be shorter.

How do you know if labour has begun?

Some women experience contractions in fits and starts at the end of pregnancy, these are slightly more intense than Braxton Hicks; will sometimes have a pattern but don't advance into actual labour. We see more "practice" labour in second and subsequent births.

Practice labour contractions

- Are usually irregular and short
- Do not progressively get closer together
- Do not progressively get stronger
- A change in activity does not change them – e.g: walking does not make them stronger
- Lying down may make them go away
- Are usually felt only in the lower belly and groin

True labour contractions

- May be irregular at first
- They become regular and longer
- They progressively get stronger
- Walking makes them stronger

- Lying down does not make them go away
- They can be felt in the front (uterus and groin) and lower back
- Having a warm bath should not make them go away

Ruptured membranes (also known as waters breaking)

Only a small percentage of women start labour with their membranes rupturing. Sometimes the membranes rupture but the contractions don't start.

Your care provider will probably have given you some guidelines about when to contact them if your membranes have ruptured.

If there are no interventions the membranes tend to rupture spontaneously during labour when the cervix is almost dilated.

No matter where you chose to birth it is wise to stay home for as long as it feels comfortable to you.

NB: Contact your care provider immediately if:

- *you have any vaginal bleeding other than the pinkish 'show"*
- *if your membranes rupture and the fluid is green in colour*

- *if you don't feel your baby move for an unusually long time*
- *or if you have constant, severe pain rather than intermittent contractions*

Mucous Plug

Throughout pregnancy, a mucus plug blocks the opening of the cervix to prevent bacteria from entering the uterus. Before labour, this mucus plug is expelled during the softening and ripening of the cervix in preparation for birth.

Somewhere in the last few days of pregnancy, you may notice a pinkish mucous discharge, which is called 'show' or 'bloody show,' as a sign that your mucous plug is being expelled. Remember though labour could be hours or even days away as the cervix gradually softens over time. If the mucous plug is lost weeks before your due date your body will generally make a new plug.

Exceptions

You may lose some, or all, of your mucous plug a little early (anything up to two weeks) in second or subsequent pregnancies because in subsequent pregnancies the cervix can ripen early and even open slightly in the last few weeks of pregnancy and so the plug becomes easily dislodged.

Sometimes the mucous plug is lost during labour and goes unnoticed.

Managing Labour Pain

During pregnancy you may start wondering/worrying about the pain that you will experience during labour and birth. Very often it is the fear of the unknown, even if this is not your first birth, because it is well known that each birth is different.

A good understanding of the labour process can be helpful to tackle this fear. This includes the understanding that there is a sense of purpose to the pain, rather than it being injury or illness. Coping skills to increase confidence and childbirth self-efficacy, ensuring that you choose the right environment (for you) and that have a good support team all play an important part in your ability to cope and how you experience the pain.

Oxytocin is the key player in the hormones of labour. It creates contractions and as it increases, it causes those contractions to get longer, stronger and closer together to ensure efficient progression of labour. On the opposing side of oxytocin are the stress hormones, which include adrenaline. Stress hormones disrupt the release of oxytocin. The more fear, tension and anxiety a woman experiences, the more pain she will feel and the more disrupted the labour process will be.

COPING METHODS

Grab the PAUSES!

The uterus contracts in waves during labour and birth. This wave has a peak and a pause. This pause is when you are able to recover and this is also when your body makes endorphins (our body's own pain relief). By relaxing each body part, physiological sighing, being quiet and calm; your body will make more endorphins and you will be more equipped to cope with the next contraction. This is a handy viscous circle which you can make full use of.

*Go to the Hormones of Labour and Birth chapter to read more -> * #chapter=qg5NUd9REy4Hv86A

Breathing

Physiological sighing

We all have the ability to tap into the power of breath as it is our single most effective tool for coping with any kind of pain or stress. The physiological sigh is quick and very effective in reducing stress in REAL TIME and it immediately helps to calm the nervous system and enables the body to make more endorphins.

You will most likely learn a variety of breathing techniques to use during contractions at childbirth classes but the physiological sigh is a great tool for **between** contractions.

It is an easy and quick 3 step breathing pattern which you can do one to three times in the pauses between contractions:

1. Take a deep inhale through your ***nose***.

2. At the end of the inhale, do another short inhale - like a quick little extra sniff of air on top of the deep inhale.

3. Slowly let all the air out through your ***mouth*** with a long extended exhale.

Acupuncture and Acupressure

According to a trial, women who received acupuncture during labour experienced less pain and required less analgesic medication.

In many countries midwives are trained to give acupuncture during childbirth and many doulas are taught acupressure techniques for pain management during birth.

Via a QR code in the bonus materials you can download a PDF with details about using acupressure during labour and birth.

Massage

Lower-back massage during a contraction can be a wonderful way to relieve pain as it works by releasing pain-killing endorphins and distracts.

Some women find that they don't want to be touched, others have a specific need for soft or hard massage or no massage movement but rather solid, counter pressure. This means that although you could practice before labour, the comfortable massage pressure will be determined by you *during* labour.

Self Hypnosis

Hypnosis is a focused state of concentration that allows you to relax your body, guide your thoughts and control your breathing. Hypnosis doesn't stop the pain of contractions. It is simply a state of mind that may help you ride the wave of each contraction and trust in your body's ability to give birth.

Self-hypnosis will aid you to let go of the fear of pain. Specialised childbirth self hypnosis techniques such as HypnoBirthing will teach you how to master this specifically for labour and birth.

Immerse yourself in warm water

Warm water diminishes stress hormones, reduces pain, eases muscular tension, helps you to relax between contractions and improves the efficiency of labour contractions. Ideally your pregnant belly should be fully immersed in the warm water but a shower can also be very effective. Studies have found that warm water immersion significantly reduces the need for pain medication -> https://evidencebasedbirth.com/water-immersion-during-labor-for-pain-relief/

Doula

A doula is a birth attendant that offers continuous physical and emotional support during childbirth. Studies have shown that women who had a doula attending their birth were less stressed, less tense, more likely to have a positive birth experience and coped far better with labour pain -> https://evidencebasedbirth.com/the-evidence-for-doulas/

TENS

A TENS (obstetric pulsar) machine works by "disturbing" pain messages from your body to your brain thereby reducing the pain. TENS also stimulates the release of endorphins. Electrical pulses are administered by four electrode pads, which are placed on your lower back and are connected to the TENS machine.

TENS machines can be hired or purchased.

Being Mobile

Most women instinctively move and sway during childbirth to help them manage the pain of childbirth. This is because it helps the baby to manoeuvre its way through the pelvis and birth canal. A mother being static or lying down makes the process slower and more painful.

Move the Mother to Move the Baby.

Bach Remedies

Bach remedies work subtly and gently to restore calm and emotional balance. They have no known side effects and can be taken before and during childbirth

Aspen: fear of unknown things.

Elm: feeling overwhelmed by responsibility.

Larch: lack of confidence.

Gorse: hopelessness and despair.

Mimulus: Fear of known things.

Mustard: Deep gloom for no known reason.

White Chestnut: mental argument, unwanted thoughts.

Walnut: helps with adjusting to change.

Rescue Remedy: for extreme or acute anxiety.

MEDICAL PAIN RELIEF

Before choosing medical pain relief it is important to have all the information about the benefits and the possible side effects in order to make an informed decision.

To choose the pain relief method or methods that are right for you, ask these following questions:

- How will it affect my birthing process and me?

- How will it affect my baby?

- What is involved in the process of administering the pain relief?

- How quickly will it work if I decide to use it?

- How long will the pain-relief last?

- Can I combine it with other methods of pain-relief?

- When during labour is the method available?

- Will I be able to feel enough to actively push my baby out?

Gas and air (Entonox)

This is a mixture of oxygen and nitrous oxide gas. Gas and air will not remove the pain, but it helps to "take you away from the pain" which makes it more bearable. It's easy to use and you control it yourself by breathing in the gas and air through a mask or mouthpiece. The gas takes about 15-20 seconds to work, so you breathe it in just as a contraction begins. It works best if you take slow, deep breaths.

Side effects and downsides of Entonox

- It can make you feel lightheaded, sick, sleepy or unable to concentrate, but if this happens you can stop using it

- It is only effective for a while; many women need to move on to other forms of pain relief if they start with gas and air too early or if their labours take long.

Pethidine

Pethidine is an opioid given either intramuscularly or intravenously. It is longer used systematically as pain relief during labour. It has significant adverse effects for mother and baby and does little more than sedate in the mother.

Side effects and downsides of Pethidine

- It can make you feel woozy, nauseous and panicked.

- It may not give you adequate pain relief.

- You will not be able to move around.

- It can suppress breathing.

- The baby will need constant monitoring.

- If pethidine is given too close to the time of birth, it affects the baby's breathing – if this happens, another medicine to reverse the effect will be given directly to the baby.

- These medicines often interfere with the baby's first feed.

Remifentanil

Remifentanil is given via an intravenous drip with a pump attached to a separate drip in the back of your hand. When you feel a contraction starting, you press a button and the pump gives you some of the medicine. Remifentanil takes up to 20 seconds to reach its full effect, so timing of pressing the button is important and can take a little practice.

Side effects and downsides of Remifentanil

- Remifentanil can make you feel sleepy, sick, dizzy or itchy.

- It suppresses your breathing and for this reason you will need to wear an oximeter on your finger to keep tabs of your oxygen levels. You may require extra oxygen.

- The baby will need constant monitoring because like pethidine, remifentanil can affect the baby's breathing after birth but also during labour because if the mother's oxygen levels are low so are the baby's.

Epidural

An epidural is considered to be the optimal method of pain relief for uncomplicated labour or non-emergency Caesarean births because it allows a woman to remain fully alert.

In most cases, an epidural gives complete pain relief.

It can be helpful if you are having a long or particularly painful labour.

An anaesthetist is the only person who can give an epidural.

How and What

In preparation for an epidural, the baby's heart rate needs to be monitored, you will receive an IV in your arm or hand and you will have a urinary catheter inserted.

An epidural is a procedure that injects a local anaesthetic into the space around the spinal nerves in your lower back. This anaesthetic blocks the pain from your labour contractions.

While you lie on your side or sit up in a curled position, an anaesthetist will clean your back with antiseptic, numb a small area with some local anaesthetic, and then introduce a needle into your back. The needle will be inserted between the bones of your spine into the space around your spinal nerves.

A small soft plastic tube will be inserted, and the needle removed. The plastic tube delivers the anaesthetic that will numb your pain.

When you have an epidural, your midwife or doctor will wait longer for the baby's head to come down (before you start pushing), as long as the baby is showing no signs of distress. This reduces the chance you'll need an instrumental delivery. Sometimes less anaesthetic is given towards the end, so the effect wears off and you can feel to push the baby out naturally.

Side effects and downsides of an Epidural

- There is an increased risk of an episiotomy and assisted delivery with forceps or ventouse.

- In about one out of hundred women, a severe, chronic headache will develop after having an epidural.

- Sometimes the epidural does not work evenly on both sides. Some women will still feel one-sided contractions.

- You will need a urinal catheter, which increases the chances of a bladder infection.

- You cannot move around.

- Your blood pressure can drop (hypotension), but this is rare because the fluid given through the drip in your arm helps to maintain blood pressure.

- The baby requires constant monitoring.
- An epidural often diminishes uterine contractions, (the body doesn't feel the pain; it thinks the birth is over and the incredible physiological, hormonal feedback loop is interrupted). This calls for augmentation and the need for Pitocin, a chemical (exogenous) form of the natural hormone, oxytocin that stimulates contractions and this can lead to a cascade of other interventions.

Nutritional Preparation for Labour and Birth

THE BODY NEEDS CERTAIN nutrients for the biological processes of softening and then dilating (opening) the cervix, sustaining efficient contractions and to help recovery during postpartum. Knowing what foods to increase or introduce is a simple way of optimising these processes.

Last weeks before your estimated due date (EDD)

Raspberry Leaf Tea

Raspberry leaf is rich in immune-boosting nutrients. It provides B vitamins, iron, niacin, manganese, magnesium, selenium, vitamin A and astringent alkaloids that nourish and contribute to the healing process postpartum.

It improves tone to the muscles of the pelvic region, including the uterus itself and is referred to as a uterine tonic.

Women through the centuries have believed red raspberry leaf tea helps to prepare the uterus for labour.

Dosage

Start with a cup a day around 34 weeks, then gradually increase to three cups as you approach your due date.

Dates

A tradition that comes from the Middle East, where it is said that women who ate dates would have easy births.

Dates contain high unsaturated fatty acids and phytoestrogens which help synthesise something called hyaluronic acid, a mediator and regulator of the cervical ripening.

Fatty acids also provide and reserve energy.

Dates are said to strengthen the uterine muscles and are rich in Vitamin K which is needed for clotting after birth.

Eat 6 dates a day from 4 weeks before your EDD.

Initiation of Labour

The pregnant body nearing birth makes prostaglandins that help to soften the cervix to ready it for dilation.

Prostaglandin production needs both the right essential fatty acids (specifically omega 6) and oestrogen. Oestrogen is a steroid hormone and cholesterol is the precursor to all steroid hormones. Without enough good cholesterol (HDL) the body cannot make steroid hormones.

Foods needed for good cholesterol production

- Coconut oil
- Eggs
- Full-fat milk products - cheese, yoghurt, cream cheese
- Butter or Ghee
- Coconut cream

Omega 6 foods

- Pine nuts
- Almonds
- Coconut
- Pecans, Brazil nuts, walnuts
- Sunflower, sesame and pumpkin seeds
- Hemp
- Dates
- Eggs
- Avocado

Hyaluronic Acid

Hyaluronic acid is also needed, together with the prostaglandins, to help to break down connective tissue of the cervix and soften the tendons and ligaments of the pelvis. The easiest way to increase dietary hyaluronic acid is to consume **bone broth**.

Efficient Contractions during Labour

Not only is **cholesterol** needed for the production of oestrogen, it is also needed to transport oxytocin to receptor cells on the uterine muscles so that the process of labour can begin and continue efficiently.

Protein

Leucine and Isoleucine are two essential amino acids found in protein foods that are needed to efficiently produce Oxytocin which is a peptide hormone, meaning it is protein based.

Sources of Leucine

- Dairy
- Beef
- Pork
- Chicken
- Tuna
- Seafood
- Pumpkin
- Seeds
- Nuts
- Peas
- Soy
- Beans

- Whey protein
- Legumes
- Sources of Isoleucine
- Meat
- Fish
- Dairy
- Eggs
- Soy
- Cashews
- Almonds
- Oats
- Lentils
- Beans
- Brown rice
- Legumes
- Chia seeds

Vitamin K

Vitamin K is essential for blood clotting and can contribute to less blood loss after birth. We need healthy gut flora to convert vitamin K1 into a usable form called K2.

K1 is the form found in plants like **parsley, kale and spinach** (difficult to absorb and needs gut flora to convert it to the usable form of K2 so that the body can absorb it.

Food sources of K2 are found in animal products like **organ meats, butter and eggs.**

Eating fermented foods will support the gut flora which in turn supports the conversion of K1 into K2 in the body. Fermented foods are sauerkraut, pickles, kimchi, tempeh, tofu, kombucha, kefir, yoghurt and miso.

Top 10 Foods in the last weeks of pregnancy

1. Bone broth
2. Avocado
3. Fermented foods
4. Butter or ghee or coconut oil
5. Sweet potatoes
6. Seeds and Nuts
7. Bananas
8. Dates
9. Meat/chicken/turkey
10. Eggs

Positions for Labour and Birth

Using different positions to stay mobile and upright during labour can help it to progress more efficiently. It can help relieve back pain, encourage your pelvis to open, and help you to cope with the pain of contractions.

It is important to realise that what may be comfortable at the beginning of labour may not be so at a later stage. Follow your instincts to find the right positions and movements for you.

Why lying down is not great

Your baby needs to descend (come down) down, onto your cervix, through your pelvis and then out through the birth canal. This means that the more upright you are, the more gravity is able to help you to manoeuvre the baby's head down.

Research has shown that women who remain mobile during labour feel more in control of the process, have more efficient labours due to effective hormonal feedback of the hormone oxytocin, which is triggered by the pressure of the baby on the cervix, which then causes the womb to contract. The contracting womb pushes the baby down creating an ever perpetuating cycle, resulting in better overall outcomes -> https://www.ncbi.nlm.nih.gov/pmc/articles/PMC4235058/

In a nutshell

- Gravity can help bring your baby down and out.

- There is less risk of compressing your large blood vessel (the aorta) that carries oxygenated blood from your heart to the rest of your body and more blood flow through the aorta leads to a better oxygen supply to the baby.

- Which leads to lowered risk of abnormal foetal heart tones.

- Which leads to a lower risk of emergency Cesarean.

- The uterus can contract more strongly and efficiently.

- The baby can get in a better position to pass through the pelvis.

- It's less painful than lying on your back.

This doesn't mean that you can't lie down on your side to rest when needed. In fact it is important to try and change your position every around every forty minutes.

Birthing positions

There is consistent evidence that when the coccyx (your tailbone) is allowed to move freely, it can move nearly 16 degrees (making more space for the baby's head to come down and out through the pelvis). In contrast, when non-flexible sacrum positions like lying back (with or without the head of the bed raised), semi-sitting up or flat on the back are used, the coccyx can only move about 4 degrees.

Flexible sacrum positions that take the weight off the tailbone are, kneeling, standing, hand-and-knees, squatting and side-lying. Birthing in water also takes the weight off the tailbone.

Standing, lean forward onto a work surface, the back of a chair, sofa, a windowsill or a delivery room or the bed (they have handy height-adjustment possibilities especially for your comfort). Put your arms around your partner's neck or waist and **lean/hang** on them.

Kneel on a large cushion or pillow on the floor and lean forwards with your head resting on your arms, on the seat of a chair.

Sit astride a chair, resting on a pillow placed across the back and top.

Sit on the toilet, leaning forwards, or sit astride facing backwards, leaning onto the cistern.

Kneel on one leg, the other bent with your foot flat on the floor.

Squat, with your partner supporting you from behind.

Walk between contractions and stop to lean during each contraction.

Use a long pole (a long window cleaning mop.) Place the pole upright and hold it quite high up with both hands while "hanging" onto it with a pulling down motion.

Hang one or two cloths/sarongs attached to strong hooks in the ceiling (if you have beams you can throw the cloths over the beams.) Make a knot in the lower end and use them to "hang" onto during a contraction. The action of pulling and hanging creates an opening, downward movement in your pelvis and helps you to relax your entire lower abdomen.

Standing and **rocking your hips backwards and forwards or in a circle** will help your baby to move through your pelvis.

Changing positions throughout labour can help to make your contractions more efficient. Allow your labour assistants to help you move into a new position every forty minutes. Their job is to keep you mobile and make you comfortable wherever you choose to be. When you are in a very strong labour, you will probably find that you don't want to move around a great deal. You'll need all your strength simply to cope with each contraction as it comes along. Don't worry, you will naturally find the position that suits you best. If you get really tired and a bed seems like the best place to be, lie down on your left hand side, because the baby gets more oxygen that way, and it can move easily into the birth canal in this position. Once you feel rested you could try to change your position again.

Positions for pushing

An upright position has gravity helping.

The combination of the muscular action of the womb, your pushing efforts and gravity is a powerful one. If the care provider prefers you to give birth on the bed, kneel on the mattress and lean against a large pile of pillows placed at the top end. Or while kneeling on the bed, put your arms around your partner's neck as he stands next to the bed so your care provider has good access to your emerging baby. You could also try squatting on the bed or on a birthing stool supported by your partner from behind.

Premature Labour

Premature labour is when labour begins prior to the 37th week of gestation.

Always alert your care provider if your membranes rupture or you have contractions before you are 37 weeks pregnant.

Placenta (the birth of)

In practice, there are three main approaches of care for the birth of the placenta.

1.

Expectant management is when the care provider waits while the uterus continues to contract after the baby is born. These contractions cause the placenta to gradually separate from the uterus and then the placenta is pushed out or birthed with the aid of gravity. Some care providers may try alternative methods (like herbs, acupuncture or homeopathy) to help the placenta to be born if it takes too long.

2.

Active management is also called "hands-on" management, where the provider uses different interventions to try to prevent severe blood loss after birth, known as postpartum haemorrhage (PPH). This management approach has come about in an attempt to reduce PPH, which is the leading cause of maternal deaths in countries defined as "low-income" by the World Bank, Surveys show that physicians are much more likely than midwives to use active management although many midwifery group practices have introduces active management into their standard care.

With traditional use of active management the care providers:

- Give an intramuscular medical form of oxytocin after the birth of the baby to help the uterus contract.

- Clamp the umbilical cord early, before the cord has stopped pulsating.

- Use controlled traction on the umbilical cord with counter-pressure on the uterus to aid the birth of the placenta.

3.

Mixed management is sometimes called "combined" management. It is a mixture of some of the components from expectant management and some of those from active management.

There are many variations, but one example of mixed management might include:

- Giving oxytocin during the pushing

- Waiting to clamp the umbilical cord until it has stopped pulsating

- Remaining "hands-off" as the birthing person expels the placenta with the aid of gravity

It is important to know that since 2019, according to the WHO, routine early cord clamping and controlled cord traction are no longer considered essential components of active management.

Natural Methods to encourage the birth of the placenta

First and foremost, ensure that the production of the birth hormones is not interrupted. Keep the mother **warm**, give her **privacy**, make sure she is **calm, no distractions** and most importantly have **mother and baby skin-to-skin** and have the mother **SMELL** her baby's head...**no bonnet on that baby!**

Acupuncture or Acupressure

If there is no acupuncturist at the birth or someone (a doula) that knows acupressure then a birth partner could try the following acupressure technique:

They sit or stand directly behind the birthing mother and apply very firm downward pressure with their fist on the top ridge of both shoulders (on the muscle, close to your neck) each time the woman has the urge to push - the acupressure point is called Gallbladder-21, Jianjing

Blowing into an empty bottle

Standing or sitting upright (if possible) blow into a large empty bottle. This will automatically put downward pressure on your pelvic floor, which could help to expel your placenta - if it is loose but not coming out.

Homeopathy Pulsatilla 30c: a single dose under the tongue

Herbs

Red Raspberry Leaf tincture may help to keep the uterus working strongly and smoothly.

Dosage

20 drops under the tongue

Vaginal Examinations

Labour is usually monitored to ensure that it is progressing as expected and one of the methods most commonly used is routine vaginal examination (undertaken at regular time intervals). Vaginal examinations are done to provide information on the position and consistency of the cervix, how dilated it is and the position of the baby.

Vaginal examinations – the origin

Historically, vaginal examinations were only done during labour to rule out complications.

The guidelines on vaginal examinations

The guidelines are a little vague on vaginal examinations and a Cochrane review ((also find more links to evidence and research under "V" in "References") concluded that there was no evidence that routine vaginal examinations done in labour improve outcomes for mothers and babies.

Evidence on vaginal examinations

Recent evidence suggests that if mother and baby are well, cervical dilation alone should not be used to decide whether labour is progressing normally. There could be something else at hand like the position of the baby or an underlying emotional issue.

Vaginal examinations are inconsistent

The measurements felt when doing vaginal examinations are subjective and inconsistent between care providers. The accuracy between practitioners is less than 50%.

Vaginal examinations can be painful and distressing

Some women find vaginal exams painful and distressing which can impact their labour process and progression due to the woman making stress hormones. It is very important to know that no one can ever put their fingers into your vagina without your consent, ever.

Vaginal examinations cannot predict the future

What the cervix is doing at the moment of a vaginal exam does not indicate what the cervix is going to do in the future. Therefore, the findings cannot effectively inform decisions about what needs to happen next such as pain medication or other interventions.

Vaginal examinations increase the risk of infection

Vaginal exams, especially done in hospital settings can increase the chance of developing an infection.

Knowing your dilation

Knowing how far you are dilated have both a negative or a positive effect on you during labour. It can be a disappointment if you have less centimetres than you hoped for but it can also be encouraging if you have more than you thought. Even though labour progress cannot be predicted purely by how dilated you are it may just be something you need to hear. Either way, you have every right to refuse or request a vaginal examination.

VBAC

A VBAC IS A vaginal birth after a previous cesarean. There are many acronyms for this phenomenon.

- VBAC = Vaginal birth after cesarean.

- BA2C or VBA3C = vaginal birth after two prior cesareans or a vaginal birth after three prior cesareans.

- TOLAC = trial of labor after cesarean.

- HBAC = home birth after cesarean

Guidelines from the Royal College Obstetricians and Gynaecologists (RCOG) in 2015 stated that a vaginal birth after a previous caesarean section has a success rate of around 75%, which is the same as for first-time mothers.

Even if the woman has had two or more previous caesareans the success rate of a vaginal birth only reduces slightly to 71%.

VBAC is a safe choice for most birthing women who have

had a C-section. If you plan on having more than one child after a previous C-section, vaginal birth may be safer than repeat C-section, which is major uterine surgery. The risks to future pregnancies and births increase with every C-section you have.

What increases your chances of a successful VBAC?

Choosing the correct care provider - know your care providers policy on VBAC

Just because a hospital room is set up to be more accommodating to birth or the care provider has promised more humanistic care, they will still be practicing obstetrics. It is their model of care. They are used to dealing with the fall out of major complications because this is their area of expertise. They also miss out on seeing physiological births which end well because this is the realm of the midwife either at home or in a birth centre. This can lead to fear-based counselling and practice and a general fear of normal birth.

Questions you can ask your care provider

- Will they insist on early induction?
- Can you move around freely during labour?
- Are they doula friendly?
- Do they have this "big baby" fear?

- Do they have a limit on the amount of time you can labour?

What else increases your chances of a successful VBAC?

- There is at least 18 months between the C-section and the planned VBAC.

- You have had a vaginal birth before.

- The reason for your last C-section is not a factor this time; for example, your last C-section happened because your baby was in a position that made vaginal birth not possible.

- You experienced some contractions - not a planned C-section

- Your labour starts on its own.

- Your labour progresses typically.

- Body work - chiropractic, Spinning Babies, pre-natal exercise.

- Emotional and mental preparation - work through any issues that may get in the way.

What reduces your chances of a successful VBAC

- You have had more than one C-section.

- You are given drugs to induce (start) or augment (strengthen or speed up) your labour.

- It has been less than 18 months between births.

- You do not have a supportive partner, family or

care provider.

- You are not fully convinced of the benefits of having a vaginal birth.
- You have not prepared for your VBAC.

In my experience both the birthing woman and her partner needs to prepare and/or other close family members who may be at the birth. It is good to be aware that the partner was most likely present at the previous birth, which may have been traumatic to witness. For a partner their priority is the safety of the woman they love and not a particular birth experience.

Waterbirth

The use of warm-water baths for labour and childbirth is used worldwide at homebirths, in birth centres and in hospital settings.

There are many benefits for both the mother and the baby.

- The effect of buoyancy that water immersion creates allows spontaneous movement of the mother.

- She moves her body according to what she feels and what the baby needs. It opens the pelvis, allowing the baby to descend.

- When a woman in labor relaxes in a warm deep bath, her body is less likely to secrete stress-related hormones. This allows her body to produce endorphins, her body's own pain relief.

- The elasticity of the perineum is increased, ensuring easier birth with fewer perineal tears.

- There is a reduced need for analgesics.

- Water eases the transition for the baby from the birth canal to the outside world. The warm liquid resembles the familiar intrauterine environment, and softens light, colours and noises.

For all you need to know about waterbirth go to Barbara Harper's informative Waterbirth website:
https://waterbirth.org/about-barbara-harper/

About Author

Jacky Bloemraad-de Boer, is a mother, grandmother, midwife, traditional Chinese medicine (TCM) practitioner / acupuncturist, nutritionist, breastfeeding counselor, herbalist, educator, holistic sleep coach and doula.

As a holistic women's health practitioner, she has provided comprehensive, integrative care and trained maternal health professionals around the world.

Her extensive experience has taught her a great deal and has left her with the belief that each maternal journey is unique and that every woman deserves to receive the kind of care which allows her to experience pregnancy, birth and motherhood as empowering and joyful.

Jacky has also written the following books in this maternal health series:

Holistic Pregnancy Manual

Holistic Postpartum Manual

ALSO BY

Also by Jacky Bloemraad-de Boer

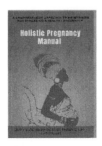
Holistic Pregnancy Manual

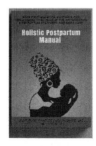
Holistic Postpartum Manual

Bonus Material

Scan the QR code for 7 Childbirth Tips

Scan QR Code for Acupressure Overview for Childbirth

REFERENCES AND RESEARCH

A

ACUPUNCTURE

Acupuncture as Pain Relief During Delivery: A Randomized Controlled Trial

https://onlinelibrary.wiley.com/doi/full/10.1111/j.1523-536X.2008.00290.x

ACTIVE MANAGEMENT OF THE THIRD STAGE

Outcomes of physiological and active third stage labour care amongst women in New Zealand

https://pubmed.ncbi.nlm.nih.gov/22188999/

B

BIG BABY

Big Baby Myth

https://pubmed.ncbi.nlm.nih.gov/18299867/

Overestimation of fetal weight by ultrasound: does it influence the likelihood of cesarean delivery

for labor arrest?

https://pubmed.ncbi.nlm.nih.gov/19254597/

BIRTHING POSITIONS

Birthing positions

Upright versus lying down position in second stage of labour in nulliparous women with low dose epidural:

BUMPES randomised controlled trial

https://www.bmj.com/content/359/bmj.j4471

The Evidence on: Birthing Positions

https://evidencebasedbirth.com/evidence-birthing-positions/

C

Midwife-led continuity models versus other models of care for childbearing women

https://www.cochranelibrary.com/cdsr/doi/10.1002/14651858.CD004667.pub5/full

Continuity of care is an important and distinct aspect of childbirth experience:

findings of a survey evaluating experienced continuity of care, experienced quality of care

and women's perception of labor

https://bmcpregnancychildbirth.biomedcentral.com/articles/10.1186/s12884-017-1615-y

D

DATES

The effect of late pregnancy consumption of date fruit on labour and delivery

https://jmrh.mums.ac.ir/article_2772.html

DELAYED CORD CLAMPING

Delayed Cord Clamping ACOG

https://www.acog.org/clinical/clinical-guidance/committee-opinion/articles/2020/12/

delayed-umbilical-cord-clamping-after-birth

Delayed Cord Clamping versus Early Cord Clamping in Elective Cesarean Section:

A Randomized Controlled Trial

https://pubmed.ncbi.nlm.nih.gov/31266035/

E

EPISIOTOMY

Episiotomies Still Common During Childbirth Despite Advice To Do Fewer

https://www.npr.org/sections/health-shots/2016/07/04/483945168/

episiotomies-still-common-during-childbirth-despite-advice-to-do-fewer

I

INDUCTION

Intrapartum intervention rates and perinatal outcomes following induction of

labour compared to expectant management at term from an Australian perinatal centre

https://obgyn.onlinelibrary.wiley.com/doi/abs/10.1111/ajo.12576

Labor induction and cesarean delivery: A prospective cohort study of first births in Pennsylvania, USA

https://onlinelibrary.wiley.com/doi/abs/10.1111/birt.12286

Ten things I wish every woman knew about induction of labour

https://www.sarawickham.com/articles-2/induction-of-labour/

Factors associated with self-efficacy in childbearing women

https://bmcpregnancychildbirth.biomedcentral.com/articles/10.1186/s12884-015-0465-8

The Facts Around Induction

https://www.aboutbirth.com.au/?m=post&category=Articles&id=101#m=post&category=Articles&id=101

P

PAIN

The Power of Pain

https://pubmed.ncbi.nlm.nih.gov/22945992/

PEANUT BALL

https://www.lamaze.org/Connecting-the-Dots/peanut-balls-for-labor-a-valuable-tool-for-

promoting-progress

PLACENTA

Myth of the ageing placenta

https://sophiemessager.com/the-myth-of-the-aging-placenta/

Birthing the placenta: women's decisions and experiences

https://bmcpregnancychildbirth.biomedcentral.com/articles/10.1186/s12884-019-2288-5?

fbclid=IwAR3u-CBhrhEYUJ6uQMcQidXD-HvKxbOGIgv2V_ppdTf21aq4-158KRjUpZJo

POSTTERM

Guidelines for the management of postterm pregnancy

https://pubmed.ncbi.nlm.nih.gov/20156009/

PRENATAL EDUCATION

Childbirth education in the 1990s and beyond

https://pubmed.ncbi.nlm.nih.gov/8791230/

PUSHING

Directed Pushing - Anterior Lip

https://midwifethinking.com/2016/06/15/the-anterior-cervical-lip-how-to-ruin-

a-perfectly-good-birth/?fbclid=IwAR2j-Y3tKIEQ-Va12HG31vBen1P-0htF_ORCiadCu4GtnGo6KDSib-Wbff3QQ

PRENATAL

https://www.medicalnewstoday.com/articles/322615#stages-of-labor

PHYSIOLOGICAL SIGH

https://www.google.com/search?client=safari&rls=en&q=physiological+sigh+breathing&ie=UTF-8&oe=UTF-8#kpvalbx=_siwsZJHCJImH9u8PwrSoeA_35

O

OMEGA 3

The mothers, Omega-3 and mental health study

https://bmcpregnancychildbirth.biomedcentral.com/articles/10.1186/1471-2393-11-46

OXYTOCIN

Oxytocin to augment and induce labor and neonatal jaundice

https://www.researchgate.net/publication/320306083_The_Effect_of_the_Use_of_Oxytocin_in_Labor_on_

Neonatal_Jaundice_A_Systematic_Review_and_Meta-Analysis

S

SPINNING BABIES

Spinning Babies

https://www.spinningbabies.com

SKIN TO SKIN

https://www.unicef.org.uk/babyfriendly/baby-friendly-resources/

implementing-standards-resources/skin-to-skin-contact/

V

VBAC

Natural Birth After A Caesarean: New Guidelines Assure Women It's 'Possible And Safe'

https://www.huffingtonpost.co.uk/2015/10/02/natural-birth-after-caesarean_n_8231566.html?ncid=other_facebook_eucluwzme5k&utm_campaign=share_facebook&fbclid=IwAR0_

G G 5 O C N Y S O 11 p L c h H 4 _ N R O r A J -
KEE0gdGXt-kHlNf36gbzzZm5KRj8how

VAGINAL EXAMS

- AIMS

https://www.aims.org.uk/information/item/vaginal-examinations-in-labour#post-heading-5

- Belly Belly

https://www.bellybelly.com.au/birth/are-cervical-checks-during-labour-necessary/

- Cochrane, Routine vaginal examinations in labour

https://www.cochrane.org/CD010088/PREG_routine-vaginal-examinations-labour

- Vaginal Examination During Normal Labor: Routine Examination or Routine Intervention?

https://www.ingentaconnect.com/content/springer/ijc/2013/00000003/00000003/art00001

- Bishops Score

https://evidencebasedbirth.com/evidence-prenatal-checks/

- Routine vaginal examinations in labour

https://www.cochrane.org/CD010088/routine-vaginal-examinations-in-labour

VEGAN

https://www.abbeyskitchen.com/nutrients-for-vegans-and-vegetarians-during-pregnancy/

WATERBIRTH

MIRACLES OF WATERBIRTH videos

https://birthpedia.net/topics/do/labor-and-delivery-prep/miracles-of-waterbirth/Waterbirth International

https://waterbirth.org/

BIBLIOGRAPHY

Zita West, *Natural Pregnancy and Acupuncture in Pregnancy and Childbirth*

Giovanni Maciocia, *Obstetrics and Gyneacology*

Verena Smidt, *Physiology in Pregnancy and Childbirth*

Dr. Gowri Motha, *Gentle Birth Method*

Michel Odent, *Primal Health*

Herbal for the Childbearing Year, Susun S. Weed

Bailliere's Midwives Dictionary

Elizabeth Davis *Heart and Hands*

Robert Bruce Newman *Calm Birth*

Arms, Suzanne. *Immaculate Deception II: Myth, Magic & Birth*. Rev. Edition. Celestial Arts, 1997.

Balaskas, Janet. *Active Birth. The New Approach to Giving Birth Naturally*. The Harvard Common Press, 1992.

Goer, Henci. *The Thinking Woman's Guide to a Better Birth*. Perigee Books, 1999.

Gaskin, Ina May. *Ina May's Guide to Childbirth*. Bantam Dell, 2003.

Harper, Barbara. *Gentle Birth Choices*. Healing Arts Press, 1994.

Noble, Elizabeth. *Essential Exercise for the Childbearing Year.*

A Guide to Health & Comfort Before and After Your Baby is Born. New Life Images, 4th Edition, 2003.

Odent, Michael. *Birth Reborn*. Second Edition. Birth Works Press, 1994.

Odent M. 1982, *Birth Reborn*, BBC Documentary video.

Scott, Pauline. *Sit Up and Take Notice! Positioning Yourself for a Better Birth*. Great Scott Publications, 2003.

Sears, William & Sears, Martha. *The Birth Book.*

Everything You Need to Know to Have a Safe and Satisfying Birth. Little, Brown and Company, 1994.

Simkin, Penny. *The Birth Partner. Everything You Need to Know to Help a Woman Through Childbirth.*

Second Edition. The Harvard Common Press, 2001.

Simkin, Penny & Ancheta, Ruth. *The Labour Progress Handbook*. Blackwell Science Ltd, 2000.

Kerstin Uvnäs Moberg, *The Oxytocin Factor: Tapping the Hormone of Calm, Love and Healing*

Manufactured by Amazon.ca
Bolton, ON